Maria Goretti Fernandes
Izabela Souza da Silva

Universal Design and the Elderly

Maria Goretti Fernandes
Izabela Souza da Silva

Universal Design and the Elderly

Vol 1. bathroom and bedroom

ScienciaScripts

Imprint

Any brand names and product names mentioned in this book are subject to trademark, brand or patent protection and are trademarks or registered trademarks of their respective holders. The use of brand names, product names, common names, trade names, product descriptions etc. even without a particular marking in this work is in no way to be construed to mean that such names may be regarded as unrestricted in respect of trademark and brand protection legislation and could thus be used by anyone.

Cover image: www.ingimage.com

This book is a translation from the original published under ISBN 978-3-330-99983-1.

Publisher:
Sciencia Scripts
is a trademark of
Dodo Books Indian Ocean Ltd. and OmniScriptum S.R.L publishing group

120 High Road, East Finchley, London, N2 9ED, United Kingdom
Str. Armeneasca 28/1, office 1, Chisinau MD-2012, Republic of Moldova, Europe
Printed at: see last page
ISBN: 978-620-5-88421-8

SUMMARY

CHAPTER 1

INTRODUCTION

The growth of the elderly population worldwide has been promoting major changes in society, mainly due to the decline in birth rates and the increase in average life expectancy rates (CARVALHO and GARCIA, 2003).

This fact is corroborated by the World Health Organization (WHO) which makes an estimate for the year 2025, where for the first time in history, there will be more elderly people than children on the planet, this growth will also occur in a vertiginous manner in Brazil, and it is reported that in 2025, the country will be the sixth country in the world in number of elderly people, with an amount greater than 30 million people (CARVALHO and GARCIA, 2003). With this, the aging population constitutes one of the greatest achievements of the century, becoming a reality for many people (PARAHYBA and VERAS, 2008). But according to the IBGE, this was only possible because the average life expectancy of Brazilians increased from 66 to 68.6 years only in the last decade.

On the other hand these data denote the need for concern with the demands, needs and limitations that accompany this new panorama as healthy ageing is an interaction between physical health, mental health, independence in daily life and social integration (SANTOS and ANDRADE, 2005), not having a standard form, being different in each individual, regardless of their chronological age.

The Brazilian legislation considers elderly the person aged 60 years or more, at this stage of life, the body undergoes a set of changes, mainly in balance, vision and hearing (CARVALHO and GARCIA, 2003), making the individual fragile, and susceptible to disabling events and with special needs.

Cultural aspects must also be observed, since speculation about human aging is as old as the history of humanity itself. In Japan, for example, those who became incapable were sacrificed, while in other ancient societies, such as China, the elderly person was considered a wise person with a prominent position among the other members. It is known that in most ancient cultures, being old meant occupying a position of prominence and privilege, but few could achieve it, since at that time life expectancy was very low. However, with the post-industrial revolution culture, ageing started to be seen only through its aspects of decadence and thus the social position of elderly individuals became secondary. In contemporary societies the elderly have occupied an inferior position, since the value of the human being is measured by the direct proportion with what is capable of being productive (BURGUESS, 1960).

Moreover, in modern society no specific role is envisaged for the elderly, abandoning them to a meaningless existence (BURGUESS, 1960), so following this same line of thought old people are considered an underprivileged minority in industrialised societies (BARRON, 1961).

In this historical and cultural context, the aging process involves other significant issues related to the physical and psychological changes of the elderly, a home for the elderly should also meet the main needs arising from the changes resulting from human aging (NÉRI, 2005).

Therefore it is necessary to include in the preparation of architectural projects environments ergonomically prepared and that follow the standards and recommended parameters. For this to happen the architectural party adopted must respect all the constraints so that it can provide the elderly, the minimum conditions for their independence, mobility, comfort and safety (SANCHES, 2010).

Therefore any housing intended for the elderly as a Long Stay Institution must offer an appropriate environment for the accommodation of these people who need a place, pleasant, safe with comfort, mobility and accessibility, properly suited to their needs, composed of environments that favor the practice of physical and leisure activities such as walking, water aerobics, gardening and even productive activities such as orchard and vegetable garden and other occupational therapies.

Thus, it is evident the need to think about the fate of this layer of society, especially in the near future, where this will be the reality of a significant percentage of the Brazilian population. Thus justifying the development of a book that meets the current needs, based on the principles of UNIVERSAL DESIGN and thus provide a better quality of life for the elderly.

CHAPTER 2

GENERAL CONSIDERATIONS ON OLD AGE

In order to gather information on the topic under analysis, a literature review was conducted to cover empirical evidence on the aging process, the functional capacity of the elderly and long-stay institutions for the elderly. In addition, the issue of ergonomics and accessibility in an architectural design for the elderly will be reported.

2.1 THE AGEING PROCESS AND ITS IMPLICATIONS FOR SOCIETIES

In the last decades of the 20th century, the increase in life expectancy brought unexpected consequences, bringing about, among others, new issues and demands from the elderly population, such as health, housing, social security, work and long-term care. These consequences also affected the family, the institution primarily responsible for the care of its dependent members, i.e., children, the elderly and the disabled. In the same period and continuing into this century, the family has also been undergoing changes in terms of the shape of its arrangements, the social division of labour among its members and its reproduction, which influences the way dependent members are cared for (HAREVEN, 1994; CAMARANO, 2002; BONGAARTS, 2001; ARRIAGADA, 2001).

It is known that these transformations began in the more developed and industrialized regions of the world and happened at different rates in different countries, and it can be said that in this first decade of the 21st century are practically universal. However, Europe took 100 years to double the proportion of older people in its population, which in developing countries such as Brazil, China and India, this should happen in no more than 20 years (LLOYD- SHERLOCK, 2004).

The reflex of these transformations is felt in the age structure, where studies point out that the top of the population pyramid widens and its base narrows, proportionally indicating an increase of the elderly in the population and fewer children and young people, in a movement which is called population aging, caused by the reduction in fertility, and by the reduction in mortality at advanced ages (CAMARANO, KANSO and MELLO, 2004).

2.2 THE AGEING POPULATION

The aging of the population is a phenomenon of global amplitude, the WHO (World Health Organization) predicts that in 2025 there will be 1.2 billion people over 60 years, with the many elderly (aged 80 or more years) constitute the age group of greatest growth. In Brazil, it is estimated that there will be about 34 million elderly people in 2025, which will take Brazil to the 6[a] position among the most aged countries in the world (SOUZA; GALANTE and FIGUEIREDO., 2003; IBGE, 2000).

These projections are based on conservative estimates as to fertility and mortality, and if there is a marked improvement in social conditions, in the poorest areas, such as the Northeast, the aging of the Brazilian population will occur in greater proportions. This can directly and significantly affect the age structure of the population and, consequently, will largely increase the problems of a given society (FREITAS, 2002).

Along with this growth, there has been a significant increase in the number of long-stay institutions, known as nursing homes. The elderly in nursing homes are doubly abandoned; first, by the family; second, by the institution itself. This double oblivion condemns them to a reality almost always identical, often defined by themselves as a daily life that is reduced to the activities of eating and sleeping. The elderly victimized by this asylum model are subjected to sedentarism, because they are not offered activities that can provide quality of life. Thus, as the population ages, the demand for long-stay institutions increases. In the United States (USA), around 5% of the elderly live in shelters which offer health, leisure and social assistance services. In England, the frequency of institutionalization is minimized through the assistance in day-hospitals, with multidisciplinary assistance to health, offered to this population, mainly in the area of rehabilitation, and these differ from the asylums and can minimize the extra work of family members of dependent elderly (CHAIMOWICZ,1998).

2.3 THE ELDERLY POPULATION IN BRAZIL

In Brazil, the total fertility rate fell from 2.7 children per woman in 1991 to 1.89 children per woman in 2008, below the population replacement level of 2.1 children per woman (DATASUS, 2009; IBGE, 2009). This means that the country is evolving towards a population with a greater number of older people.

For this reason the characteristics of the Brazilian elderly were gathered from the national report on the ageing of the Brazilian population. This document is one of the most complete documents ever produced on the subject, with broad participation from state bodies and civil society entities. In it, the ageing of the Brazilian population is evidenced by an increase in the participation of the contingent of people over 60 years of age from 4% in 1940 to 9% in 2000. Moreover, the proportion of the population aged over 80 has increased, altering the age composition within the group itself, which means that the population considered elderly is also ageing. This group represents the fastest growing population segment, although it is still a small contingent: from 166,000 people in 1940, the group of elderly people rose to almost 1.8 million in 2000, representing 12.6% of the elderly population in 2000 and approximately 1% of the total population (IBGE, 2000).

In Brazil, the phenomenon of ageing can be exemplified by an increase in the participation of the population over 60 years of age in the total national population from 4% in 1940 to 8% in 1996. Moreover, the proportion of the "older" population, i.e. those aged 80 and over, is also increasing, altering the age composition within the group itself, that is, the population considered to be elderly is also ageing. This leads to a heterogeneity of the so-called elderly population segment (CAMARANO, 2002).

Several scholars report that in the period from 1980 to the year 2000, parallel to a total population growth of 56%, it is estimated an increase in the elderly population in Brazil of more than 100%. The age group aged 60 years or over will rise from 5% of the total population in 1960 to 14% in 2025, when Brazil will have a proportion of elderly people similar to that of developed countries (COELHO FILHO and RAMOS, 1999). Figure 1 shows the projection of aging in Brazil for the period 1991 to 2050 (IBGE, 2000).

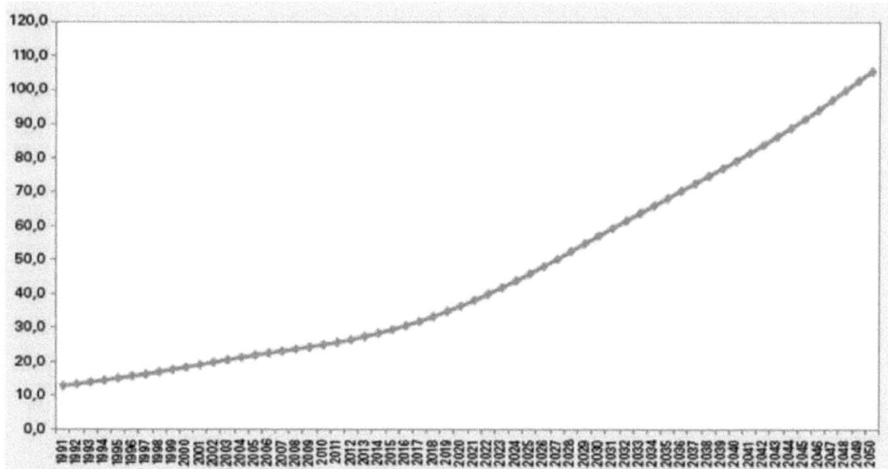

Figure 1: Projection of ageing in Brazil from 1991 to 2050 Source: (www.ibge.gov.br) Accessed in: May 2011.

2.4 THE AGEING PROCESS AND ITS CONSEQUENCES FOR THE ELDERLY

Population ageing is one of the greatest achievements of this century. Being able to reach an advanced age is no longer a privilege of a few people. In contrast, many societies are not consistent with these demographic changes, in the following sense: they attribute values related to competitiveness to their groups, value the ability to work, independence and functional autonomy, among others. In reality, many of these beliefs and values, can not always be accompanied by the elderly, if we take into account some changes and losses that are often associated with old age. It is observed that these beliefs are built in the form of representations, in the daily conversations of the groups of the elderly (VELOZ; NASCIMENTO e CAMARGO, 1999).

According to Chaimowicz (1998), the elderly population, is expected to face increasing difficulties such as:

1) the non-existence of social policies to support caregivers, with regard to family members or other individuals who provide direct assistance to the elderly in their basic activities, namely: food, home help, medical assistance and guidance services, among others;

2) the size of families in Brazil, which has been decreasing due to the fall in fertility;

3) the increase in the proportion of marital separations, elderly people living alone, couples choosing not to have children, and mothers raising their children alone;

4) elderly residing with relatives whose total income does not exceed three minimum wages;

5) and finally, the formal support system that has not been able to replace the role of the family .

These difficulties associated with the health problems inherent to aging bring great consequences to the elderly population. However, there is no standard way of ageing, which is specific to each individual, regardless of their chronological age. This physiological process is a complex event, where biological and socio-cultural conditions are strictly related. In this way, the alterations of the aging process can make the elderly individual more fragile and susceptible to incapacitating events, among them falls (SANTOS and ANDRADE, 2005).

It is important to highlight that during aging there is a set of progressive and differential degradation processes that the body undergoes after its developmental phase, emphasizing in three modalities: balance, hearing and vision (DARÉ, 2006). With age the movements become slower, the reaction times of an elderly woman are longer than those of a young adult, and this difference tends to grow in more complex tasks which require the capacity of discrimination between several different stimuli. The vision gradually loses its efficiency, with a decrease in the visual acuity, accommodation capacity, dark adaptation and colour vision (GUIMARÃES; OLIVEIRA; MORAES, 2009).

However, ageing cannot be seen only as a process of reduction of capacities and the emergence of health problems, but rather as a process in which skills are lost and others are developed, in an accumulation of experiences and competences, which will allow life to have a meaning that is not static, always having to be fulfilled, that is, it is never definitive (SANTOS apud DARÉ, 2006).

On the other hand, due to the lifestyle adopted by some people and hereditary factors, some people reach old age with a gradual loss of health. This loss of health is somehow perceived by the elderly, but the occurrence of accidents can anticipate restrictions and drastically change their life picture. He becomes passive or completely dependent on third parties, suffers physical constraints due to his own difficulties, whether inside or outside home. This occurs due to alterations promoted by the reduction of balance, vision and hearing, the elderly population develops difficulties in the handling of equipment used in the domestic environment, thus generating a relationship of dependence and a lack of freedom, being obliged, in the course of their lives, to leave their homes, thus causing a decrease in their quality of life (DARÉ, 2006).

2.4 FUNCTIONAL LIMITATIONS AND ENVIRONMENTAL FACTORS IN FALLS IN THE ELDERLY

It is known that during the aging process the elderly may develop serious functional limitations, such as difficulties in walking, lack of coordination and balance, which may lead to frequent falls in daily life. Associated to these facts are the environmental factors which also contribute to falls in the elderly. Falls in the elderly arise due to functional limitations inherent to the aging process and it has been observed that many falls occur at home, where some environmental factors may play an important role in up to half of all falls in the elderly. Among these factors one can highlight: inadequate lighting, slippery surfaces, loose carpets with folds, high or narrow steps, obstacles in the way (low furniture, small objects, wires), the absence of handrails in corridors and bathrooms, excessively low or high shelves, inadequate shoes, and or foot pathologies, mistreatment, excessively long clothes, among others (PEREIRA; FERNANDES e SANTOS , 2007).

On the other hand, the decrease in the effectiveness of motor strategies of body balance that affect the elderly and the functional unbalance are one of the main factors that limit the life of the elderly. However, it is worth pointing out that falls are not only related to factors considered risk related to the individual. Associated to postural instability imbalance, there is a multifactorial component external to the physical function, among which are the ergonomic adaptations which may modify the risk of falls in persons with compromised mobility. These are important, considering that most falls tend to occur in the elderly home itself, having the physical environment as the cause. The indexes of this incident are multiplied in elderly people living in Long-Stay Institutions (LTCF), as these mostly lack adaptations or, when present, are introduced in an inadequate manner (FABRÍCIO; RODRIGUES e COSTA JUNIOR, 2004).

2.5 THE ISSUE OF THE INSTITUTIONALISATION OF THE ELDERLY

It is quite significant the effect of advanced age added to certain conditions causing dependence which are very frequent among the elderly, namely dementia, hip fractures, strokes, rheumatological diseases and visual impairments are the most common problems. These situations also reduce the individual's ability to overcome environmental challenges (CALDAS, 2003). Therefore, many elderly people with functional complicatons are institutionalised in nursing homes or geriatric homes.

The main causes that lead elderly people to settle in nursing homes were described by Born and Boechat (2006) as being:

a. Family problems;
b. Health problems;
c. Limitation of activities of daily living;
d. Mental Situation;
e. Ethnicity;
f. Lack of social support;
g. Poverty, among others.

However, it is worth noting that most of these older people were taken to the institutions by family members and that some went there on their own initiative (ROLIM, 2002).

2.6 HISTORICAL ASPECTS OF ASYLUM INSTITUTIONS

Asylums for the elderly have not appeared recently. It is known that Christianity was a pioneer in caring for the elderly. History reports that the first asylum was founded by Pope Pelagius II (520-590 AD), who turned his house into a hospital for the elderly (ALCÂNTARA, 2004).

The term asylum comes from the Greek asylos and the Latin asylu. The word asylum is defined as a house of social assistance where poor and destitute people, such as beggars, abandoned children, orphans and the elderly, are gathered for sustenance or education. The asylum is also considered a place where those who come to it are exempted from the enforcement of laws, and this environment is still related to the idea of guardhouse, shelter and protection of the place. This idea occurs independently of its social, political character or care with physical and/or mental dependencies, because the generic character of this definition appeared to denominate places of assistance to the elderly as, for example, shelter, home, rest house, geriatric clinic and nursing home. In the current days it looks for to standardize the nomenclature, it has been proposed the denomination of institutions of long permanence for elderly (ILPI), defining them as establishments for integral attendance to the elderly, dependent or not, without family or domiciliary conditions for its permanence in the community of origin (SBGG, 2003).

Historically, there are some facts that are related to the issue of asylums, as for example in Colonial Brazil, the Count of Resende argued that old soldiers deserved a dignified and "rested" old age. But it was only in 1794, in Rio de Janeiro, that the Invalids' Home appeared, not as a charity action, but as recognition to those who had rendered service to the motherland, so that they could have a peaceful old age (ALCÂNTARA, 2004).

The history of old people's homes is similar to that of hospitals, as in their beginning both sheltered elderly people in situations of poverty and social exclusion. In Brazil, the first institution for the elderly was built in Rio de Janeiro in 1890 and was called Asilo São Luiz para Velhice Desamparada. The emergence of this asylum promoted a greater visibility to the issue of old age (GROISMAN, 1999).

In this context, institutionalisation was a world apart and entering it meant breaking ties with family and society. The situation was much worse when there were no specific institutions for the elderly, who were sheltered in beggars' asylums, together with other poor, mentally ill, abandoned children and the unemployed. It was only at the end of the 19th century that Santa Casa de Misericórdia de São Paulo, an entity that promoted assistance to beggars, due to the increasing number of admissions for the elderly in this location, started to define itself as a geriatric institution in 1964 (BORN, 2002).

2.7 NURSING HOMES AND THE ISSUE OF ECONOMY OF CARE

Nursing homes or long-stay institutions (LTCF) for older people provide long-term care. Long-term care is defined as a set of health, social and personal services provided for a continuous period of time to people who have lost or never had a certain degree of functional capacity (Mc CULLOUGH, 2002). Such care falls within the growing care economy developed in recent decades. The care economy is understood as an economy of services provided for the well-being of others (BLOCK, 2003) and this occurs within the family or institutional environment.

Currently, the caregiver is classified as family or formal caregiver. Family or informal caregiver is understood as any person who defines him/herself as a caregiver, providing unpaid support for at least four hours a week to a person over 65 years old, at home or even in a residential care setting. However, this definition does not exclude carers outside the circle of kinship, for example, friends and neighbours. It includes anyone who provides unpaid assistance to meet the needs of an older person in terms of health, personal care, transportation, emotional and psychological support, home care, administration or financial support. Formal caregiver includes the service organization provided by third parties who provide financial support by providing companionship and care to people with special needs (LAMURA *et al.*, 2008).

It is worth noting that recent changes in the structure of the family, the primary repository of care responsibilities for dependent members (children, the sick, the disabled and the elderly), have raised questions about the appropriateness of continuing to attribute the provision of these services mainly to the family. As male and female roles have evolved within the family, in the labour market and in civil life, the institutional arrangements that have predominated in care work over the last century have proved in need of revision (SILBAUGH, 2001).

A large part of this care economy, structured throughout the 20th century, is difficult to measure, since it is part of the informal care provided in general by women. As Block (2003) argues, informal care is not included in the Gross Domestic Product of nations, for example, but it is slowly gaining visibility. On the other hand, the provision of formal care services, including long-term care provided in specially designed residential institutions, called Long-Term Care Facilities, has been on the rise.

On the other hand, the range of long-term care has expanded, and is not restricted to care provided in institutions. In the first decade of the 21st century, efforts in several countries, such as the United States, Germany, Denmark, England, among others, were aimed at providing care for the elderly in their homes, and there was a proliferation of alternatives, such as day centres or night centres, professional home care services, both for personal care and health care. It is also observed in these countries the adoption of support policies such as the inclusion of home care, paid rest for informal caregivers, as it occurs in Germany and Japan, the inclusion of informal caregivers in social security, as in Japan. (GIBSON *et al.*, 2003; KITCHENER and HARRINGTON, 2007; CAMARANO, 2005a; TELLECHEA, 2005; BATISTA *etal.*, 2008).

On the other hand, the recent focus of research on informal caregivers aims to alleviate the pressure that the prolonged care of an elderly person represents for families.

This pressure is considered a determining factor in the early admission of the elderly person to a long-stay institution. The Madrid Plan of Action on Ageing of 2002 (LAMURA ET AL.2008) recommends that caregivers should be a key factor in the early admission of the elderly to an institution.

Importantly, a study of the experiences of family carers of older people in using support services has been carried out. This work was carried out in 2003 with six European countries (Sweden, Germany, UK, Poland, Italy and Greece). These countries formed a working group to carry out comparative research on the issue of informal care for the elderly and the support they receive from public authorities. In 2004, information was collected on the availability, use and acceptance of care support for families in these countries, with the aim of better targeting policies on this topic, adjusting them to the real needs of caregivers. This information was collected through questionnaires applied to 1,000 caregivers in each country who devoted at least four hours a week to the care of older people, thus obtaining comparable empirical evidence of the experiences, difficulties and preferences reported by family caregivers in Europe in the use of support services (LAMURA ET AL.,2008).

2.8 CHARACTERISATION OF LONG-STAY INSTITUTIONS

The Long Stay Institutions (LTCF) when they are intended for elderly people are called Long Stay Institutions for the Elderly. These institutions are different from hospitals and consist of collective residences, with cohabitation rules and operating logic that varies according to their public. Often they take care of people with physical and cognitive frailties in various degrees of severity. Other times they offer only residence and shelter (KITCHENER and HARRINGTON, 2004).

Despite all the initiatives and efforts to keep the elderly as long as possible in their own homes, it has been observed that the new alternatives of prolonged or permanent care in families and communities do not replace, in certain situations, Long-Stay Institutions for the Elderly. Although institutional care is not predominant in most of the countries where information is available, the number of residents is not negligible: in France in 1998, 500,000 of the 12 million elderly people resided in long-term care facilities, which represented 4.1% of the elderly population. Norway is the OECD country with the highest percentage of older people being cared for in institutional care homes: 11.8%, while the rate of formal residential care was 15.6%.14 Denmark, meanwhile, is the OECD country with the highest rate of formal residential care for older people (21.0%). There the percentage of older people residing in institutional care homes was 9.1% in 2000. In developed countries, no more than 12% of the elderly live in institutional care facilities and that the proportion of elderly people cared for in institutions is always much lower than those cared for in their homes, with the exception of the UK, where the proportions are similar (GIBSON, M.; GREGORY, S.; PANDYIA, S., 2003).

The organisation of long-term care for the elderly population is happening with the multiplication of care programmes for the elderly in the community and in their homes, which enable them to remain in their own homes until a more advanced age, Long-stay Institutions tend to be more sought after by older individuals, with considerable functional losses and dementia syndromes (BORN and BOECHAT, 2006; DESESQUELLES and BROUARD, 2003).

At the time when a reduction in the rate of residence in institutional care homes was indicated, from the 1980s onwards, Canada effectively presented a decrease in the number of hospitalizations of individuals under 85 years of age. But it did show an increase of around 18% in the demand for institutions as a result of the increase in the proportion of people over 85 in the population. The same result was found in the United States, where, in 1985, only 1.3% of seniors aged 65 to 74 years resided in nursing homes, compared to 22% in the range of 85 years or more (BORN and BOECHAT, 2006). Today, with the advancement of medicine, preventive care and the improvement of living conditions, especially in developed countries, life expectancy without disabilities increases and they are postponed to increasingly advanced ages (GIBSON, M; GREGORY, S.; PANDYIA, S., 2003).

As generally occurs in developing countries, also in Brazil there is no habit in families of resorting to LCIs as an alternative of long-term care for the elderly (UN, 2002). Camarano (2007) estimated 103,000 elderly residents in homes for the elderly in 2000, representing only 0.8% of the total population. Despite the low proportion of elderly residents in homes for the elderly in Brazil, it seems that the number of long-stay institutions for the elderly has increased since the 1990s, as pointed out by data from the IPEA Research on Operating Conditions and Infrastructure in Long-Stay Institutions for the Elderly, still in the field. This inference is made using data on the year the institutions were founded, a variable collected by the Research (CAMARANO, 2007). In the four regions where the data is already consolidated, 48.1% of the existing LTCIs were created after 1990. Similarly to findings in other countries, in Brazil, residents aged 80 years or more are the largest group of residents in long-term institutions. The first results of the IPEA Research point this out for the four researched regions: 34,0% in the North (CAMARANO, 2007), 23,6% in the Centre-West (CAMARANO, 2008), 42,1% in the Northeast (CAMARANO, 2008b) and 34,5% in the South (CAMARANO, 2008a).

2.9 THE GENERAL CONTEXT OF LONG-STAY INSTITUTIONS FOR THE ELDERLY (ILPIS) IN BRAZIL

In Brazil, there is no national survey on institutions for the elderly (BORN, 2002). But there is a study of the French sociologist Hôte, conducted in 1984, this work investigated the programs for the elderly in Brazil, where it was observed from 0.6% and 1.3% of the elderly residing in institutions asylums. In countries like Brazil, with extreme socio-economic inequality and cultural diversity, the care of the elderly assumes different outlines. For example, in the south and southeast of the country, where the purchasing power is greater, institutionalisation tends to be similar to that of developed countries.
However, there are still many elderly people institutionalised due to chronic degenerative diseases and or the impossibility of the family to maintain them (CAMARANO, 2005).

Regarding the regulatory issues of nursing homes, the resolution of the collegiate board of directors of ANVISA / RDC No 283 of 26 September 2005, which approves the Technical Regulation establishes the operating standards for Long-Term Care Institutions for the Elderly in Brazil. This resolution defines such institutions as governmental or non-governmental institutions, of residential character, destined to the collective domicile of people with age equal or superior to 60 years, with or without family support, in condition of freedom, dignity and citizenship. This is a rather generic definition, which leaves room for several interpretations and does not eliminate the confusion and ambiguity that proliferates both in literature and in legal documents. Such confusion goes beyond the linguistic use of the expression and extends to the definition of the purpose and nature of these institutions, of residence, provision of health services or social assistance.

The family situation of the elderly in Brazil reflects the cumulative effect in socio-economic, demographic and health events along the years, demonstrating that the size of the offspring, the separations, the celibacy, the mortality, the widowhood and the migrations, originate, in the development of the decades, types of familiar and domestic arrangements, where to live alone, with relatives or in nursing homes, can be the result of these dislocations. Most of the time, nursing homes usually arise spontaneously from the social needs of the community, and in this case, problems occur in the quality of life that the residents find there (LOUZÃ ET AL., 1986).

Thus, the main existing services offered to this population are directed to health, being common, in most of the capitals of the country, private or philanthropic asylum institutions directed to the elderly, and, with rare exceptions, those maintained by the State. In Brazil, although a large proportion of institutionalised elderly people are dependent due to physical or mental problems, poverty and abandonment are the main reasons for institutionalisation, and the majority, especially in the metropolitan regions. These asylums are inappropriate and inadequate homes for the needs of the elderly, which do not offer them social assistance, basic hygiene care and food. Furthermore, these places also hinder interpersonal relationships in the community context, which are indispensable to maintain the elderly for life and for the construction of their citizenship. They also constitute the oldest and universal form of care for the elderly, outside of their family environment, having, as an inconvenience, to promote their isolation, their physical and mental inactivity, thus having negative consequences on their quality of life (ROLIM, 2002).

However, Decree No 1.948 of July 3, 1996, emphasizes in Article 3 °, that the institution asilar has the purpose to meet, on a boarding school regime, the elderly without family ties or without conditions to provide their own subsistence, in order to meet their needs of housing, food, health and social interaction. Law 8.842, January 1994, in article 4, paragraph III, also gives priority to the elderly care provided by their families, instead of the asylum system. However, with the existence of several factors, such as demographic, social and health, lead to increased demand for institutionalization (LOUZÃ ET AL., 1986).

As for the characteristics of nursing homes for the elderly, they are usually places with space and physical areas similar to large living quarters. Rare are those that have specialised staff for social and health assistance or that have a work proposal aimed at keeping the elderly independent and autonomous. They live, most of the time, as if they were in reformatories or boarding schools, with rules for entering and leaving, few possibilities for an active social, affective and sexual life. In reality, many times what is found are deposits of people, who, based on the idea of love for the neighbour and support to the homeless, consider that the shelters, together with the care provided to them, are sufficient to people who are in their last days of life (DAVIM *et al.*, 2004).

It is difficult to know how many institutionalised elderly people there are in Brazil. According to the government data, today there are around 19 thousand elderly assisted in asylums. The number can be much higher if we take into account that many of the institutions of this type are not registered and many others work, effectively, in the underground (ROLIM, 2002)

2.10 ERGONOMICS AND ACCESSIBILITY IN THE CONTEXT OF SPACE INHABITED BY THE ELDERLY

To understand nursing homes and their limitations regarding environmental, ergonomic and accessibility factors present in the space inhabited by the elderly, it is necessary to understand the aspects related to the home-space interface and universal design.

2.11.1 HUMAN-SPACE INTERFACE AND UNIVERSAL DESIGN

Since ancient times man has been concerned with the relationship between the inhabited space and his own body. In the 1st century BC, the Roman architect Marcus Vitruvius Pollio, known as Vitruvio, wrote a complete treatise on architecture in ten books, called *Arquitectura*, where he studied the proportions of the body and their metric implications. Euclid, a Greek mathematician from the 2nd century BC, founder of the Alexandrian School, called the "metrical and extreme ratio" the division of a segment into two parts following a defined proportion. But in the XIX century these 2 parts became known as the Golden Section, which today is present in any study of size and dimension related to the human body (BARROS, 2000).

In the Renaissance, Leonardo da Vinci , conceived his famous drawing of the human figure, based on Vitruvio's man, and on mathematical studies involving the Golden Section, imagining man in harmony with the universe. In 1946, the Swiss-French architect Le Corbusier (1887-1965), created a model of harmonic standards of dimensions to the human scale, applicable to Architecture and to the Industrial Design, called by the author Modulor , which made the approximation between the metric system used in France and Germany and the English system, of inches, used in England and United States. Thus, the Modulor started to determine heights and widths for the performance of several domestic and work activities, being widely adopted by architects and industrial designers (BARROS, 2000).

Universal design is another aspect used by architects in the projection of spaces. This concept of Universal Design was developed among professionals in the area of architecture at the University of North Carolina - USA, with the aim of defining a design of products and environments to be used by everyone, to the greatest extent possible, without the need for adaptation or specialized design for people with disabilities. Thus, the idea of universal design is to create accessible products for all people, regardless of their personal characteristics, age or abilities. These universal products accommodate a wide range of preferences and the individual or sensory abilities of users. The goal is that any environment or product can be reached, manipulated and used, regardless of an individual's body size, posture or mobility. It is important to report that the Universal Design is not a technology directed only to those who need it, because its principle is precisely to ensure that everyone can use safely and autonomously the various built spaces and objects (CARLETTO and CAMBIAGHI, 2011).

In 1987, the American Ron Mace, an architect who used a wheelchair and an artificial respirator, created the terminology *Universal Design.* Mace believed that it was not the birth of a new science or style, but rather a perception of bringing together the things we design, making them usable by all people. But in the 1990s, Ron himself created a group with architects and advocates of these ideals to establish the seven principles of universal design. These concepts are globally adopted for any full accessibility program and are defined as : egalitarian, adaptable, obvious, known, safe, effortless and comprehensive (CARLETTO and CAMBIAGHI, 2011).

a) Equalitarian: That which is destined for equal use. These are spaces, objects and products which can be used by people with different abilities, making all environments equal.

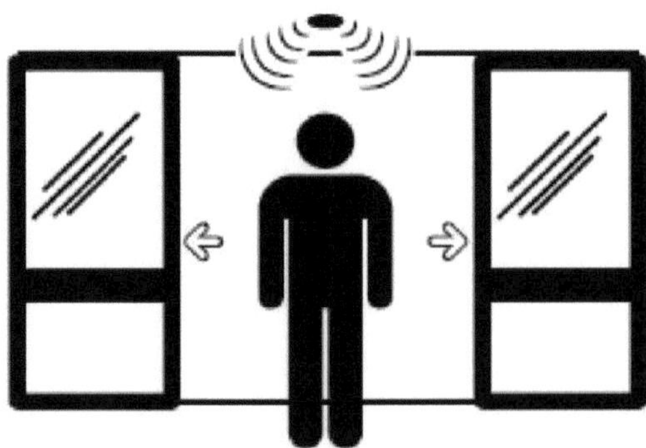

Figure 2 - Doors with sensors that open without requiring physical strength or reach of the hands. Source: Carletto and Cambiaghi, 2011.

b) Adaptable: The one that is intended for flexible use. Product design that caters for people with different abilities and diverse preferences, being adaptable to any use.

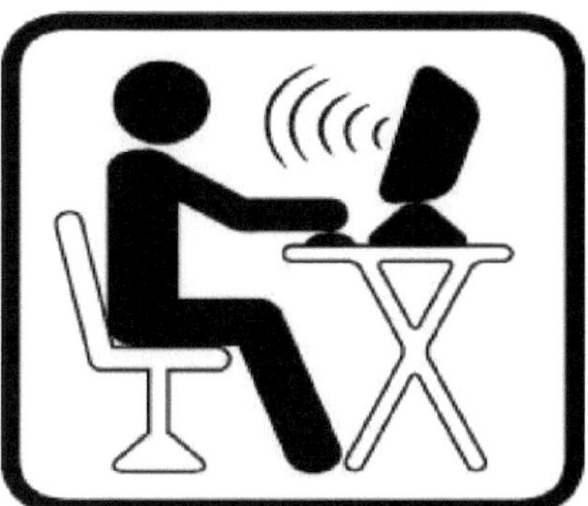

Figure 3 - Computer, keyboard and mouse with programmed "Dosvox" type.
Source: Carletto and Cambiaghi, 2011.

c) Obvious - Those with simple and intuitive usage, which are easy for anyone to understand, regardless of their experience, knowledge, language skills or level of concentration.

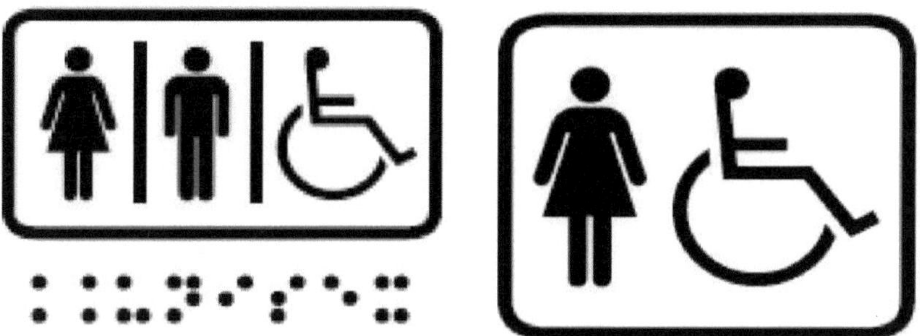

Figure 5 - Symbols and raised letters, Braille and auditory signalling.
Source: Carletto and Cambiaghi, 2011.
Figure 4 - Toilets for women and people with disabilities.
Source: Carletto and Cambiaghi, 2011.

d) Known - Easily Perceived Information. When the necessary information is transmitted in a way that meets the needs of the receiver, be it a foreigner, visually or hearing impaired person.

e) Safe: Error-tolerant. Designed to minimise the risks and possible consequences of accidental or unintended actions.

f) Effortless - They must present low physical effort to be used efficiently, with comfort and minimum fatigue.

g) Comprehensive - Division and Space for Approach and Use. Which establishes appropriate dimensions and spaces for access, reach, manipulation and use, regardless of body size (obese, dwarf, etc.), posture or mobility of the user (people in wheelchairs, with prams, walking sticks, etc.).

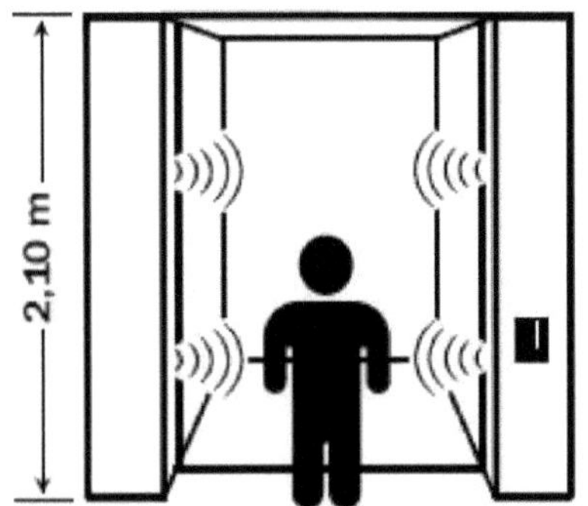 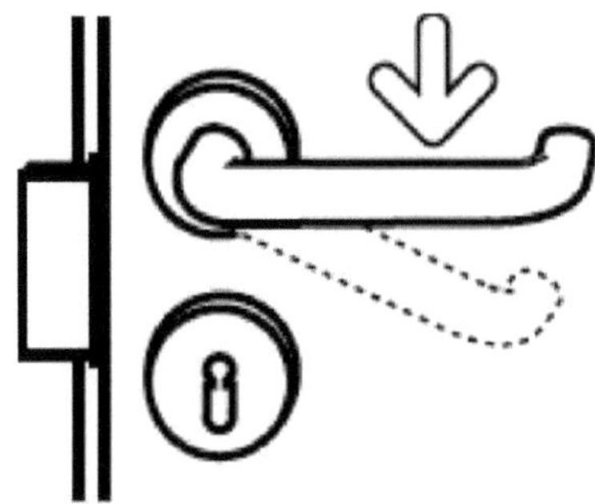

Figure 6 - Elevator with sensor, so that the door is not closed in the middle of the procedure.
Source: Carletto and Cambiaghi, 2011.
Figure 7 - Lever handle is easier to handle.
Source: Carletto and Cambiaghi, 2011

Based on these principles it is necessary to make use of a universal design for buildings, as it proposes to idealise spaces that are designed to meet a wide range of the population, considering variations in size, sex, weight or different abilities or limitations that people may have. The four principles of the Universal Design of accessibility are: to accommodate individuals with different standards and situations; to reduce the energy expenditure required to use products in the environment; to make environments and products more understandable to the disabled and to think of products and environments as systems, in order to improve the service to people with disabilities (SANTOS ; SANTOS and RIBAS, 2005)

Acting this way it is obtained environments that meet the proposals of universal design, without, however, costing more. The degree of accessibility required for a certain construction depends on its nature, but there is a basic requirement that is the same for all built facilities: it must be accessible for people (OLIVEIRA, 2003).

2.11.2 THE ELDERLY WITH SPECIAL NEEDS

Currently in Brazil and worldwide, thousands of people with some kind of disability are being discriminated against in the communities where they live, or even having their access to their professional career hindered (MACIEL, 2006). For when we approach the subject regarding the "correct" terminology to be used when discussing disability, this often becomes a topic of discussion in the society in which we live (MEDEIROS and DINIZ, 2001)

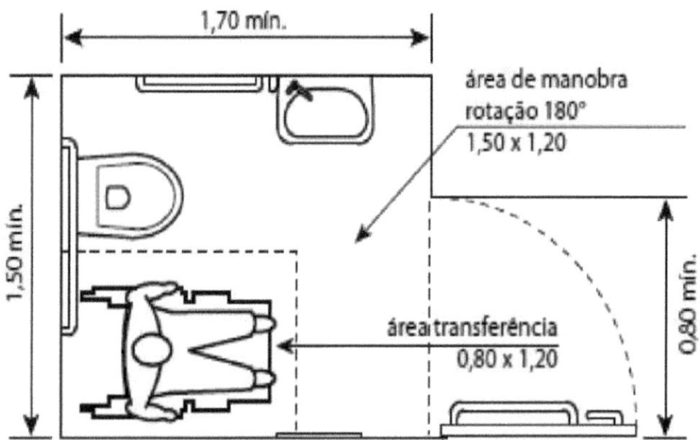

Figure 8 - Toilets adequately sized for people in wheelchairs or who are with babies in their prams.
Source: Carletto and Cambiaghi, 2011.

It should be remembered that the term people with special needs (PNE's) includes obese people, elderly people, autistic people, gifted people, people with learning difficulties, people with organic insufficiencies, conduct problems, attention disorders (such as hyperactivity), obsessive compulsive disorder, emotional disorders and mental disorders. PNE's are also people with disabilities, which is represented by the loss or abnormality of a psychological, physiological or anatomical structure or function that generates incapacities for the development of activities within the normality standard for human beings in this context the

The elderly is a person with special needs and deserves greater security in their home environment (VASCONCELOS and FERNANDES, 2008).

For some time, the use of the term disabled to refer to persons experiencing disability was avoided, as it was believed to be a stigmatizing term. From this situation, alternatives were sought which could more adequately describe the nomenclature linked to it, such as, for instance, person with special needs, person with disability, or the most recent, person with disability. All of them seeking primarily to highlight the importance of the person when referring to disability (MEDEIROS and DINIZ, 2001).

According to the IBGE census carried out in 2000 and the results of a recent survey in Brazil, there are 24.5 million people with some kind of disability. Of this number, 2% are regularly employed, 52% are inactive and, of the latter, 29% live in poverty. Among the disabilities presented by the participants of the census, motor, hearing, mental and visual disabilities stand out. The geographical distribution of the disabled, the highest percentage regards the Northeast region, where the following states stand out: Paraíba (18.7%), Rio Grande do Norte (17.6%), Piauí (17.6%), Pernambuco (17.4%) and Ceará (7.3%). And, lower percentages can be found in the other states of the national territory, as for example in São Paulo (11.3%), Roraima (12.5%), Amapá (13.2%), Paraná (13.5%), and the Federal District (13.4%) (FRANÇA; PAGLIUCA e BAPTISTA, 2008).

However, building an inclusive society requires changing ideas and practices that have been built over time. One of them refers to the importance of providing care and support to the family and the community, so that people with special needs (PNEs) have better living conditions, within their limitations. This fact is also related to the elderly. The Ministry of Health is responsible, since the 1988 Constitution, for the commitment to restore the model of care in Brazil, starting from a referential of health as citizenship rights, assuming the organisation of increasingly resolute, comprehensive and humanised services. Regarding the families of PNEs, it is possible to highlight that they have been in a position of dependence on professionals in different areas of knowledge, in order to receive guidance on how to proceed with the special needs presented by their relatives, making it necessary to clarify them well, as well as establish management skills of such situation within the family environment, this includes the necessary ergonomic adaptations for the promotion of functional independence of the elderly (CARVALHO and SOUZA, 2009).

2.11.3 ACCESSIBILITY FOR ELDERLY PEOPLE WITH SPECIAL NEEDS

Accessibility is the possibility and condition of reach for the use with safety and autonomy of buildings, public spaces, furniture and urban equipment. This presupposes freedom of choice or individual choice in the act of relating to the environment and to life. Basing oneself on the idea that people with disabilities depend on the help of others generates embarrassing situations which only perpetuate segregation (ABNT, 1994). The purpose of accessibility is to allow a gain of autonomy and mobility to a wider range of people, even to those who have reduced mobility or difficulty in communicating, so that they may enjoy the spaces with more safety, confidence, comfort (PRADO, 1997).

The Brazilian Association for Technical Standards (ABNT) presents a set of standards, through NBR 9050, whose objectives are to establish the criteria and technical parameters to be observed when designing, constructing, installing and adapting buildings, furniture, urban spaces and equipment to accessibility conditions (ASSOCIAÇÃO BRASILEIRA DE NORMAS TÉCNICAS - ABNT, 2004).

Cities are places where people live together. Individuals work, live, socialise and circulate in them, and therefore they must be accessible to all. Public spaces in cities are usually created for an idealized standard of individuals, this standard excludes people with disabilities. There is a huge unpreparedness of the places to offer adequate access conditions to those who have difficulties in locomotion (CORDE, 1997), this situation clearly happens with the elderly, especially when they have some kind of disability and need places with accessibility.

Adapting the environments used, such as homes, workplaces, hospitals, clinics and offices, shops, leisure areas and other places regularly visited, means allowing, in addition to the right to come and go and the guarantee of equality, a modern conception of approaching the theme of disability, which is the current trend. The correct adaptation of the internal environments and the minimum necessary spaces used in the buildings, as well as, the reform and adaptation of the furniture and equipment most used by the user, acquiring the maximum of his/her independence is defined as the standard ideal condition (MOREIRA, 2000).

Architectural Barriers - impediment of accessibility, natural or resulting from architectural or urbanistic implantations (ABNT, 1994). They are obstacles which impede or bring limitations to the access, freedom of circulation and movement of people. The barriers are divided into urbanistic architectonic barriers (exist in public roads and public spaces); architectonic barriers in the buildings (exist inside private and public buildings); architectonic barriers in the transportation (exist in the means of transportation). Examples of architectural barriers are: stairs for access, narrow doors and circulation, small lifts which do not have Braille signalling, non-adapted toilets and inadequate service counters. And as an example of urban barriers, one may cite the following: unevenness or inadequate coverings on pavements which make it difficult for the disabled to move about, unevenness between the curb and the roadway in places used for crossing, narrow pavements with inadequate pavement and obstacles which make it difficult for the visually impaired to detect them, lack of parking spaces in car parks for the disabled, absence of urban furniture, such as, for instance, public telephones, mailboxes at a height which is inadequate for persons using wheelchairs (CORDE, 1997).

2.11.4 ERGONOMICS AND THE ELDERLY

Ergonomics is the study of the relationship between man and his work, equipment and environment and particularly the application of knowledge of anatomy, physiology and psychology, in solving the problems arising from this relationship (IIDA, 2001), but this science can be used not only in the organization of workstations. It also includes the anthropometric adequacies of the measures of furniture, the correct arrangement of equipment and environmental conditions. It is easy to realize that the ergonomic intervention is global and able to act as adjuvant in preventing falls in the elderly and improving the physical environment, through an effective ergonomic planning (FERNANDES ET AL., 2009)

The elderly, especially those with special needs, also benefit from the use of ergonomic adaptations, whether in the work or home environment. The ergonomic organization of this home can significantly interfere in reducing the likelihood of falls in this population (VASCONCELOS; FERNADES e SIQUEIRA, 2008)

2.11.5 ERGONOMIC ADAPTATIONS FOR ELDERLY PEOPLE WITH SPECIAL NEEDS

It is known that Ergonomics is an important instrument in everyone's life, because it is a necessary tool in the promotion of effectiveness, comfort and economy of physical energy in the daily life activities of the population (CORREA; ANTUNES; MERINO, 2003). In this way it is pertinent the applicability of ergonomic knowledge in order to evaluate and establish a diagnosis that can guide the creation of safer and more appropriate environments for people (SÁ, 2006).

Regarding PNEs, it is not enough to carry out excellent professional rehabilitation programmes when there is no preparation of the home and work environments to receive them. To make adaptations that make the execution of professional and usual activities feasible, becomes fundamental for the effectiveness of the placement, at work and in society, for these people. There are many ways to facilitate the daily routine of PNEs, these initiatives originate in domestic activities, where it is possible to facilitate the internal access of the house, the reach of objects, the presence of ramps, lifts, and adequate transportation (NAKAMURA, 2003; PEREIRA; FERNANDES e SANTOS, 2007).

However, there are few built spaces, environments or products that consider the perceptual, psychic, cognitive, biomechanical, and anthropometric characteristics of the elderly population. Therefore, the primary importance in emphasizing a greater attention to the characteristics of this population, proposing ergonomic improvements in their environments. (MARTINS e CANTO, 2001)

Showing the relationship between ageing and disability is important for several reasons, firstly because ageing is accompanied by some limitations in physical and sometimes intellectual abilities; secondly, because interdependence and care are not something necessary only in exceptional situations, but rather ordinary needs at various times in people's lives. Third, because of the predictability of ageing, it is pertinent to understand that much disability is the result of a social and economic context that reproduces itself over time, since disability in old age is partly the expression of inequalities that arose in the past and are maintained until current times (MEDEIROS and DINIZ, 2001).

2.11.6 THE ELDERLY WHEELCHAIR USER

The investment in ergonomic adaptations is essential to ensure the right to come and go with autonomy, independence, safety, and the opportunity for social participation. It is necessary to raise awareness and mobilize society in search of actions that promote accessibility and social inclusion of people with disabilities or reduced mobility (MUNIZ,

2005; BRITO et al, 2006).

In this context, elderly wheelchair users must receive special attention, as their needs interfere in the whole project of the building, and all anthropometric measures of reach must be observed, as well as the needs of the user/chair set for their displacements, reach to doors, windows, cabinets, benches, activating devices, etc, so that the minimum conditions of independence and comfort are met. (SANTOS; SANTOS e RIBAS, 2005)

In order to design accessible buildings for elderly wheelchair users, it is essential to consider ergonomic criteria for the displacement and use of the built space and equipment. The best strategy to unite the principles of ergonomics and architecture, is to enable the early performance of the responsible professionals, in other words, that they are working together from the moment of the construction of the project, until its full realization and use by the user, as for example, the spaces of the room and the bathroom of the elderly. (ELY, 2003)

2.12 ERGONOMIC PLANNING FOR THE ELDERLY

The ergonomic planning in environments designed for elderly people involves the adaptations in the spaces used by these people. Thus, the elderly bedroom and bathroom deserve special attention.

2.12.1 ADAPTATIONS IN THE ROOM AND BATHROOM FOR ELDERLY PEOPLE WITH SPECIAL NEEDS

The quality of life of the elderly can be maximized when they feel safe in their home environment and, as such, enjoy functional independence. As the bedroom and the bathroom are the places of greatest activity of the elderly, these should be planned or adapted to their special needs, mainly due to age-related sensory alterations that hinder their free access to these spaces.

2.12.2 THE ROOM OF THE ELDERLY WITH SPECIAL NEEDS

The greater susceptibility of the elderly to falls is due to the current functional decline of the aging process, such as the increase in reaction time and the decrease in the effectiveness of motor strategies of body balance. As a result of this, imbalance becomes one of the main factors that limits the life of the elderly (SÁ et al, 2006)

Also according to these authors, the causes of falls in the elderly may be varied and associated. The factors responsible for them have been classified in the literature as intrinsic and extrinsic. Among the intrinsic factors it is possible to highlight those resulting from physiological alterations related to aging, diseases and effects caused by drugs. And, among the extrinsic factors, those factors that depend on social and environmental circumstances that create challenges to the elderly.

Considering that the home environment is the place where the elderly remain for most of the day, it is essential that these environments are properly organized and adapted to meet all their needs, also promoting safety, comfort and functional convenience. Therefore, in relation to the elderly room shown in figure 9, it is important to carefully observe doors, windows, handles, switches, height and arrangement of rooms and objects, adapting them according to ABNT/NBR 9050, and taking into consideration the opinion and priorities established by the user and his family. In figure 9, we find the adequate dimensions for the elderly patient's room, where it is necessary to have manual and visual reach, a 0.80 cm door entrance, and a 0.90 cm width for the elderly to be able to manoeuvre to the bathroom, bed and cupboards.

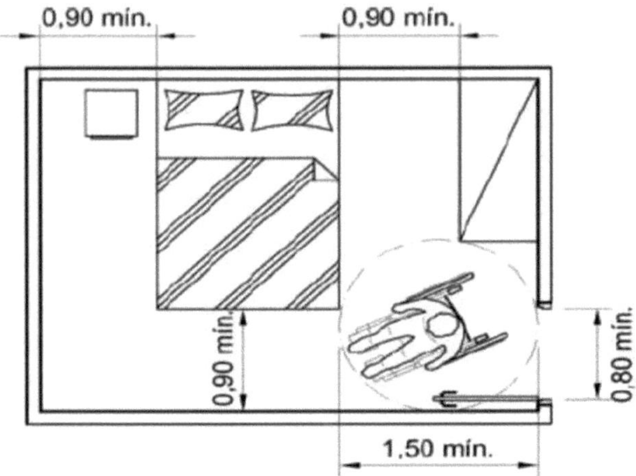

Fig. 9 - Appropriate dimensions for the elderly wheelchair user's room. Source: ABNT (2004)

2.12.3 THE TOILET FOR OLDER PEOPLE WITH SPECIAL NEEDS

The bathroom is the most dangerous room in the home for the elderly because it is a wet environment, because its floor is more slippery, because it has glass walls, worktops or shelves, because it has sharp edges and little space for movement (STAMATO and MORAIS, 2007).

The boxing also continues to be a highly commented upon place within this environment, due to the need for non-slip flooring, safety bars, support benches and mats with suction cups inside, these authors also reveal.

Other authors emphasize the need for specific accessories in the bathroom to facilitate access for people with disabilities. Such examples are: support bars for transference, protection for the lavatory, reservation of enough space for wheelchair rotation (Figure 10), height of the toilet bowl, and adaptations in the pit, mentioned in the previous paragraph (ABNT, 2004; QUALHARINI and ANJOS, 1997).

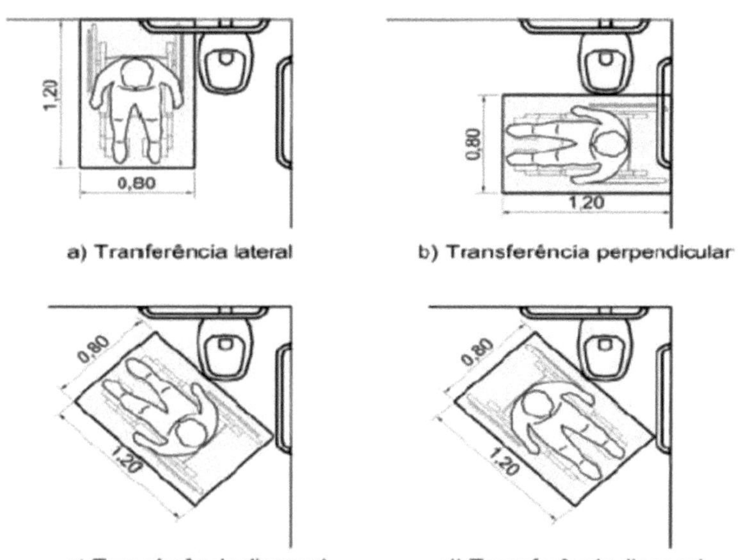

Figure 10 - Several types of transfer with the wheelchair in the bathroom enabling the rotation of the chair. Source: BRASIL (2004).

Two support bars shall be installed on the side wall of the seat, one vertical and one horizontal, or alternatively, a single "L" shaped bar, complying with the following parameters: the vertical bar must have a minimum length of 0.70 m, at a height of 0.75 m from the finished floor and at a distance of 0.45 m from the seat's front edge; the horizontal bar must have a minimum length of 0.60 m, at a height of 0.75 m from the finished floor and at a maximum distance of 0.20 m from the seat's anchorage wall and the "L" bar, replacing the vertical and horizontal bars, with bar segments of 0.70 m minimum length, at a height of 0.75 m from the finished floor in the horizontal segment and at a distance of 0.45 m from the seat's front edge in the vertical segment. (Figure 11) (NBR-9050)

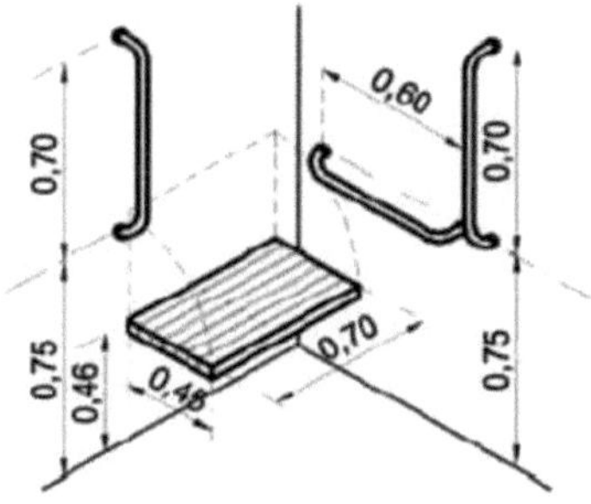

Figure 11 - Boxing perspective with the support bars.

When the structure of the sink is taken into consideration, a frontal approach area must be provided, extending to at least 0.25 m underneath it. Figures 12 and 13 show the approach area with support bars for the sink (NBR 90-50).

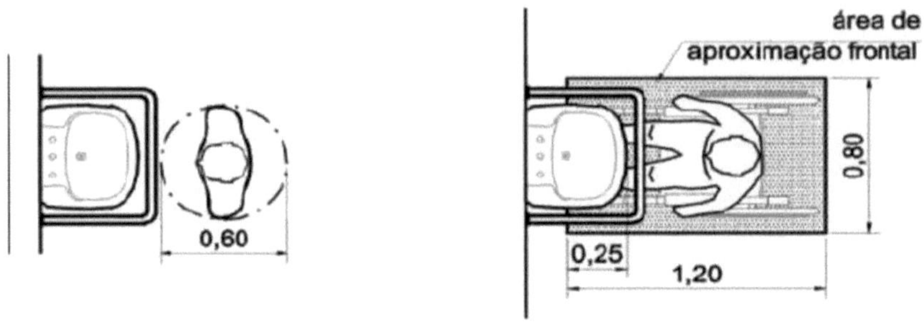

Figure 12 - Approach area with support bars.
Source: ABNT (2004).

Suspended urinals must be located at a height of 0.60 m to 0.65 m from the front edge to the finished floor. The flush actuation, when present, must be at a height of 1.00 m from its axis to the finished floor, require light pressure and be preferably of the lever type or with automatic mechanisms. It is recommended that the human actuation force be less than 23 N. The urinal must be equipped with vertical support bars, fixed at a distance of 0.60 m, centered by the axis of the piece, at a height of 0.75 m from the finished floor and minimum length of 0.70 m. (Figure 14) (NBR 90-50)

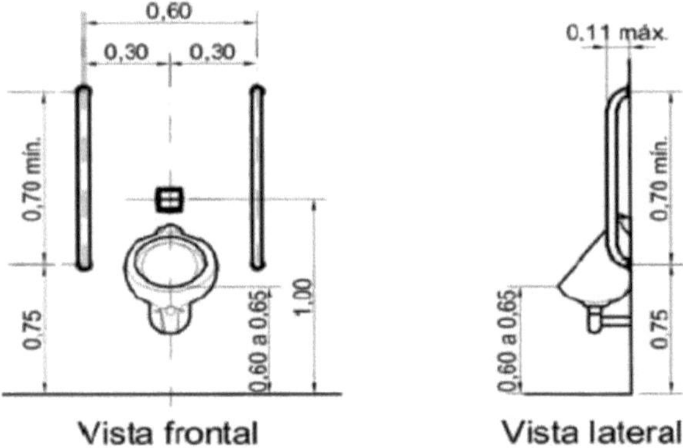

Figure 14 - Fontral and side view of the urinals.
Source: ABNT (2004)

Toilet accessories such as coat hangers, soap dishes and towel racks must have their area of use within the comfortable range according to figure 15 (NBR 90-50).

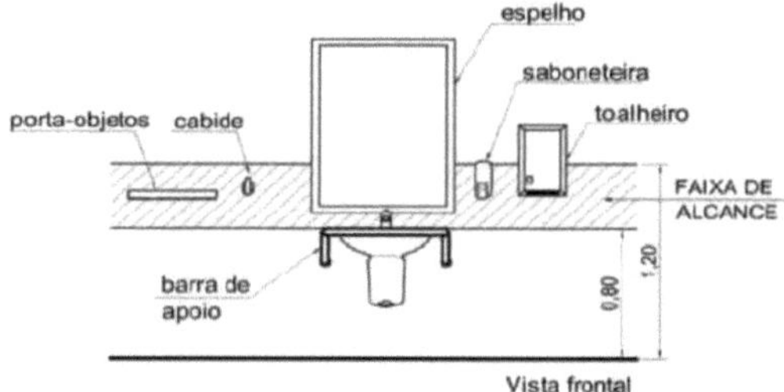

Figure 15 - Accessories next to the washbasin. Source: ABNT (2004)

The built-in paper bins or those that extend up to 0.10 m from the wall must be located at a height of 0.50 m to 0.60 m from the finished floor and at a maximum distance of 0.15 m from the front edge of the basin.

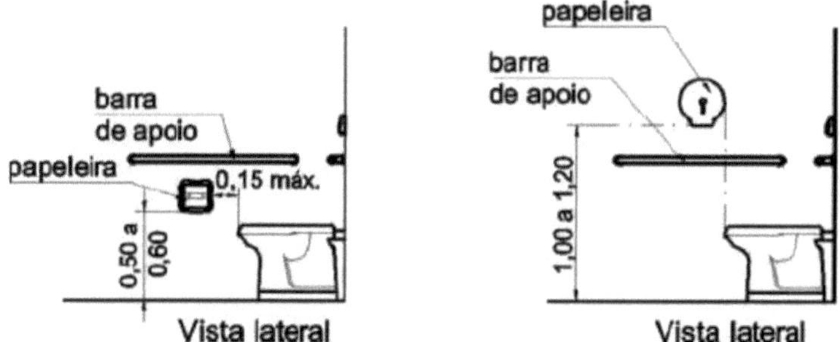

Figure 16 - View of Embedded and Non-Built-in Paper Frames. Source: ABNT (2004)

Figure 17 shows a door model according to NBR 90-50. The doors must be able to be opened with a single movement and their handles must be of the lever type, installed at a height between 0.90 m and 1.10 m. When located in accessible routes, it is recommended that the doors have in their lower part, including the door jamb, a coating resistant to impact caused by canes, crutches and wheelchairs, up to a height of 0.40 m from the floor (NBR90-50).

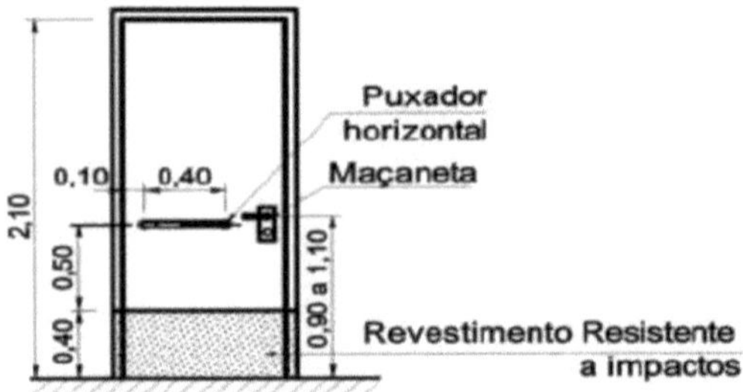

Figure 17 - Doors with lining and horizontal handle.
Source: ABNT (2004)

Handrails shall be between 3.0 cm and 4.5 cm wide, without sharp edges. A free space of at least 4.0 cm must be left between the wall and the handrail. They should allow good grip and sliding and preferably have a circular section as shown in figure 18. (NBR 90-50)

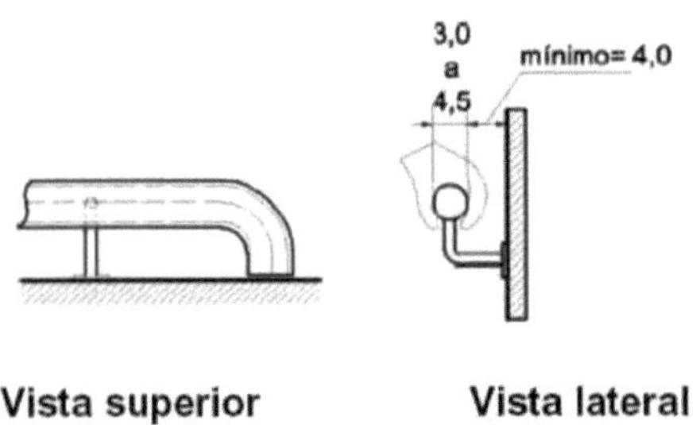

Figure 18 - Handrail grip.
Source: ABNT (2004)

Professionals who have knowledge of age-related sensory changes and environmental modifications should take on the role of advisors. Providing information to architects and designers will increase safe access to the home for the elderly. Encouraging architects and builders to incorporate universal concepts that allow structures to be adaptable to accommodate age-related sensory changes may be best suited to promote an improved quality of life for the elderly (GUCCIONE, 2002).

The location of the support bars must meet the following conditions: They must be close to the toilet bowl, on the side and at the bottom, horizontal bars for support and transfer must be placed, with a minimum length of 0.80 m, at 0.75 m height from the finished floor (measured by the fixing axes). The distance between the basin axis and the side bar face to the vessel must be 0.40 m, with this bar positioned at a minimum distance of 0.50 m from the front edge of the basin. The bottom wall bar shall be at a maximum distance of 0.11 m from its external face to the wall and extend at least 0.30 m beyond the bowl axis towards the side wall.

If it is impossible to install bars on the side walls, hinged or fixed side bars (fixed to the back wall) are allowed, provided that the appropriate safety and sizing parameters are observed, and that these and their supports do not interfere in the turning and transfer area. The distance between this bar and the basin axis must be 0.40 m, and its end must be at a minimum distance of 0.20 m from the basin front edge.

In the case of basins with a close coupled box, the installation of the bar on the bottom wall must be guaranteed in order to prevent the box from being used as a support. The minimum distance between the underside of the bar and the lid of the coupled box must be 0.15 m as shown in figure 19 (NBR 90-50)

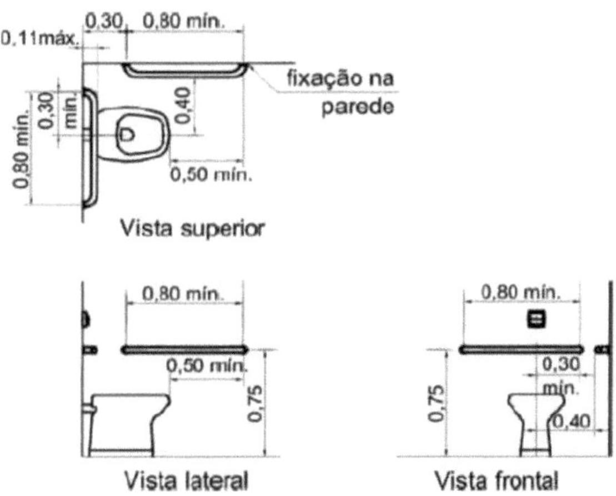

Figure 19 - Sanitary basin - Side and bottom support bars.
Source: ABNT (2004)

The sanitary basins must be between 0.43 m and 0.45 m above the finished floor, measured from the top edge, without the seat. With the seat, this height must be a maximum of 0.46 m. The installation of a pedestal at the base of the basin must follow the projection of the basin base and not exceed 0.05 m of its contour (Figure 20) (NRB 90-50).

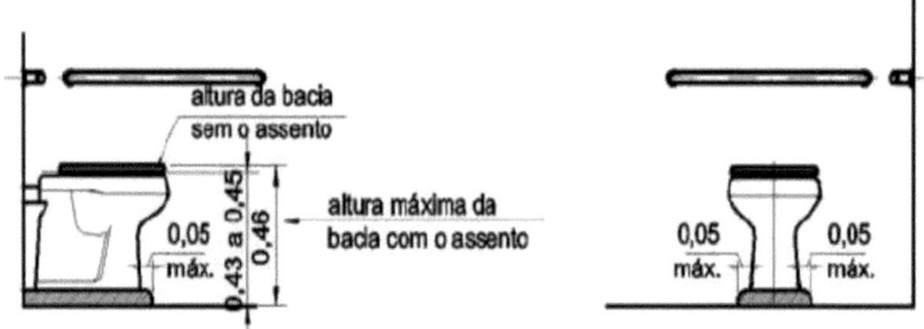

Figure 20 - Height adaptation of the sanitary basin with a pedestal. Source: ABNT (2004)

The discharge drive must be at a height of 1.00 m from its axis to the finished floor, and preferably of the lever type or with automatic mechanisms (Figure 21) (NBR 90-50)

Public toilets and changing rooms must allow one person to use all sanitary parts (Figure 22) (NBR 90-50).

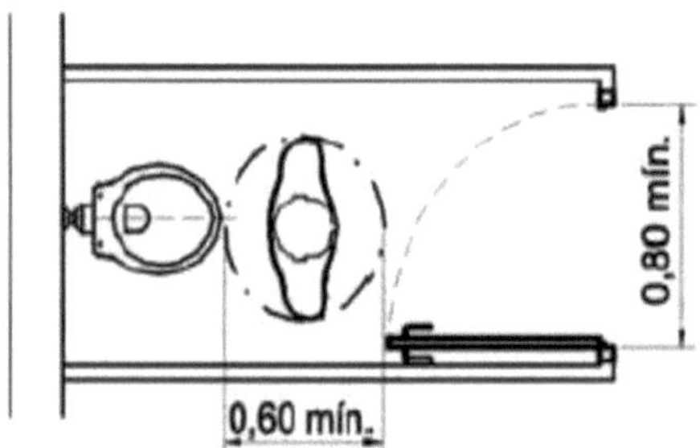

Figure 22 - Boxing with door opening inwards.
Source: ABNT (2004)

It is known that living at home and interacting with the home environment can be a challenge for the elderly individual. This challenge becomes even greater when the elderly person has special needs. To solve this problem, there must be a balance between functional capacity and adaptation to the environment in order to promote strategies to minimize the impact of these difficulties on the functional independence of the elderly (GUCCIONE, 2002).

It is essential to correlate that the suggestions presented in this work regarding the ergonomic adaptations that should be performed in the room and bathroom of elderly individuals with special needs are cited by several authors and scholars on the subject. This is because for an elderly individual to live independently, he/she must be able to safely perform a complement of personal care activities and home control. The specific nature of the activities required by a given individual depends on many variables. For the elderly to live independently, they need to perform ADLs (activities of daily living) and maintain control of their basic personal hygiene and survival needs. Home environments such as the bathroom and bedroom are places where the elderly perform their functional activities, such as mobility in bed, getting in and out of bed to the chair, bathing, using the toilet, dressing, grooming, these activities are sometimes called personal activities of daily living.(SONN et al., 1996)

Ergonomic adaptations and assistive devices can be used to facilitate the performance of ADLs, for example, using the seat in the shower to facilitate bathing. (MEANS et al., 1996)

The greater susceptibility of the elderly to suffer falls is due to the functional decline resulting from the aging process, such as the increase in reaction time and the decrease in efficacy of motor strategies for body balance. Imbalance is one of the main factors that confine the life of the elderly. However, falls are not only related to factors considered risk related to the individual. Associated to unbalance due to postural instability, there is a multifactorial component external to the physical function, among which are the ergonomic adaptations which may modify the risk of falls in persons with compromised mobility. These are very important, considering that most falls tend to occur in the elderly home, having the physical environment as the cause. The indexes of this incident are multiplied in elderly people living in Long Stay Institutions (LTCI), once most of them lack adaptations or, when present, are introduced in an inadequate manner (FABRÍCIO, RODRIGUES e COSTA JUNIOR, 2004).

As half of the falls occur indoors, it is necessary to adapt the house to the elderly, just as it is done to prevent risk situations for domestic accidents involving children. The other half of the falls occur in public spaces, where urban policies for accessibility are required, in order to make it easier for the elderly and physically challenged people to move around. The bathroom is one of the residential rooms considered most dangerous for the elderly, mainly because they are the wet room in the house and therefore have a slippery floor; also because they are composed of walls, doors, countertops or glass shelves, because there is the use of many sharp and cutting objects inside these rooms, for both have gas equipment for the use of fire, for the fact that their furniture has sharp edges and limited space for movement and performance of activities inherent to these rooms and etc. (STAMATO, 2007)

According to ABNT/NBR 9050 the minimum dimensions of the boxes should be 0.90m by 0.95m. The boxes must have a hinged or removable bench with rounded corners and a non-slip waterproof surface, a minimum depth of 0.45m, a height of 0.46m from the finished floor and a minimum length of 0.70m. They must also be provided with vertical and horizontal support bars. On the wall where the seat is fixed, a vertical bar shall be installed with a height of 0.75m from the finished floor and a minimum length of 0.70m, at a distance of 0.85m from the side wall of the seat, where two support bars shall be placed, one vertical and the other horizontal, obeying the following parameters, the vertical one shall have a minimum length of 0.70m, height of 0.75m from the finished floor and distance of 0.45m from the frontal edge of the seat; the horizontal must have a minimum length of 0.60m, height of 0.75m from the finished floor and distance of 0.20m from the wall where the bench is fixed (BRASIL, 2002).

Other authors report that the prevalence of falls among elderly people in nursing homes occurs in about 38.3%. These falls are more common in the asylum environment (62.3%), being the room the environment where the highest number of falls occur. This study was a cross sectional design carried out with the participation of elderly individuals aged 65 years or older, living in nursing homes for elderly people in the city of Rio Grande, RS, in 2007. Included in the study were the nursing homes, old people's homes and geriatric clinics registered in the Health Surveillance of the city, a total of 15 old people's homes in 2005. (GONÇALVES et al., 2008)

According to the Statute of the Elderly (2003), in the chapter that deals with housing, institutions that house elderly people are required to maintain housing standards compatible with their needs. A study carried out in nursing homes in the city of João Pessoa/PB, sought to study the relationship between the built environment and the quality of life of the individuals who live in them. The results pointed out that the architectural errors found in the institutions studied suggested a reflection on the way these elderly people are treated. For, besides living in conditions of social exclusion, they began to have the environment in which they live as a potentializer of diseases, whether physical or emotional. (TOMÉ e MÁSCULO, 2006)

CHAPTER 3

BIBLIOGRAPHIC REFERENCES CONSULTED

ALCÂNTARA, AO. Velhos institucionalizados e família: entre abafos e desabafos. Campinas: Alínea; 2004.149 p.

ARRIAGADA, Irma (ed.). Familias latinoamericanas. Diagnóstico y políticas públicas en losinicios del milenio, in Revista de la CEPAL N° 57 - Serie Políticas Sociales, Social Development Division, December 2001, Santiago, Chile, pp. 17-30.

ASSOCIAÇÃO BRASILEIRA DE NORMAS TÉCNICAS - ABNT. NBR 9050: Acessibilidade a edificações, mobiliário, espaços e equipamentos urbanos. Rio de Janeiro, 2004.

BARRON, M.L. The Aging American. New York: Thomas and Crowel, 1961

BARROS, C.F.M. Casa segura: uma arquitetura para a maturidade. (2000).
BARROS. C.F.M. Casa segura - Uma arquitetura para a maturidade. Ed. Armazém digital. Available at: < http://www.casasegura.arq.br > Accessed on: 09 Apr. 2011.

BATISTA, Analía Soria; JACCOUD, Luciana de Barros; AQUINO, Luseni; EL-MOOR, Patrícia Dario. Envelhecimento e Dependência: Desafios para a Organização da Proteção Social. Brasília: MPS, SPPS, 2008.

BLOCK, Fred. The 'Thing' Economy and the 'Care' Economy. Alternet, 2003. Available at http://www.alternet.org/story/17146 accessed 11 May 2008.

BONGAARTS, J. Household Size and Composition in the Developing World. Population Studies Nov 2001; 55 (3):263-79.

BORN, T. Cuidado ao idoso em instituição. In: Papaléo Neto M, et al, organizadores. Gerontologia. São Paulo: Atheneu; 2002. p. 403-13.

BORN, Tomiko, BOECHAT, Norberto Seródio. A qualidade dos cuidados ao idoso institucionalizado. In: FREITAS, Elizabete Viana de (org.) Tratado de Geriatria e Gerontologia. 2ª ed. Rio de Janeiro: Guanabara Koogan; 2006. pp.1131-1141.

BRASIL. ANVISA - National Health Surveillance Agency Resolution - RDC No. 50, of 21 February 2002.

BRITO, L. S. et al Acessibilidade de cadeirantes em clínicas de fisioterapia do Plano Piloto de Brasília - DF. Universitas: Health Sciences, Brasília, v. 4, n. 1/2, p. 1735, 2006.

BURGUESS, E. W., Introduction, In: Burguess, E. W. (Org.), Aging in Western Societies, Chicago: The University of Chicago Press, 1960.

CALDAS, C. P.. Aging with dependence: responsibilities and demands of the family. Cad. Saúde Publica, Rio de Janeiro, v. 19, n. 3, p. 733-81, may/jun. 2003.

CAMARANO, A. A. Envelhecimento da população brasileira: Uma contribuição demográfica. Rio de Janeiro: IPEA, 2002. Available at: <http://www.ipea.gov.br/pub/td/2002/td_0858.pdf>. Accessed on: 11 feb. 2009.

CAMARANO, Ana Amélia (coord.), Características das Instituições de Longa Permanência para Idosos: região Sul. Brasília: IPEA, 2008a. pp.138.

CAMARANO, Ana Amélia (coord.), Características das Instituições de Longa Permanência para Idosos: região Nordeste. Brasília: IPEA, 2008b. pp.348.

CAMARANO, Ana Amélia et al. Idosos brasileiros: indicadores de condições de vida e de acompanhamento de políticas. Brasília: Presidência da república, Subsecretaria de Direitos Humanos, 2005.

CAMARANO, Ana Amélia, KANSO, Solange, MELLO, Juliana Leitão e. Como vive o idoso brasileiro? In: CAMARANO, Ana Amélia (Org.) The new Brazilian elderly: far beyond 60? Rio de Janeiro: IPEA, 2004.

CAMARANO, Ana Amélia. A. Instituições de longa permanência e outras modalidades de arranjos domiciliares para idosos. In: NERI, Anita L. (org.) Idosos no Brasil: vivências, desafios e expectativas na terceira idade. São Paulo: Fundação Perseu Abramo, Edições SESC SP, 2007. pp. 169-190.

CAMARANO, Ana Amélia. Envelhecimento da População Brasileira: uma Contribuição Demográfica. In: FREITAS, Elizabete, et al. Tratado de Geriatria e Gerontologia. 1ª ed., Rio de Janeiro: Guanabara Koogan , 2002, v. único, c. 6, p. 58 - 70.

CARLETTO, ANA CLAUDIA; CAMBIAGHI, SILVANA. The Primer "Universal Design - A Concept for All". Available at: ttp://www.maragabrilli.com.br/desenho- universal.html accessed on 05 June 2011.

CARVALHO, J. A. M.; GARCIA, R. A. O envelhecimento da população brasileira:um enfoque demográfico. Cad. Saúde Pública, Rio de Janeiro, v. 19, n. 3, p. 725-733, mai-jun. 2003.

CARVALHO, T. J.; SOUZA, T. S. Programa Itinerante de Educação e Saúde: Qualidade de

Vida na famílias de pessoas com necessidades especiais. Em Extensão, Ituitaba, v. 8, n. 1, p. 91-104, jan./jul. 2009.

CHAIMOWICZ F. Os idosos brasileiros do século XXI: demografia, saúde e sociedade. Belo Horizonte (MG): Postgraduate; 1998.

COELHO FILHO, J. M.; RAMOS, L. R.. Epidemiologia do envelhecimento. Rev. Saúde Publica. São Paulo, v. 33, n. 5, p. 445-53, oct.1999.

CORDEIRO, A. D. A Construção de uma caminhar mais seguro para o idoso: o Design de uma bengala ergonomicamente adequada. In: CONGRESSO BRASILEIRO DE ERGONOMIA, 14, 2006. 14th Congress. Curitiba: ABERGO, 2006. 3p.

CORRÊA, A. R., ANTUNES, J. R. P., MERINO, E. A. D. Estudo ergonómico de acessibilidade para a população idosa: o caso do jardim botânico de São Paulo. [S.I.]: Fisionet, 2009. Available at: <http://www.fisionet.com.br/monografias> Accessed on 03/01/2009.

CULLEN, Gordon.Urban Landscape. Architecture and Urbanism. Lisboa: year 1983 Edições 70.

DARÉ, A. C. The perception of the elderly of the domestic environment: an inclusive process. In: CONGRESSO BRASILEIRO DE PESQUISA E DESENVOLVIMENTO EM DESIGN, 7, 2006, Paraná. 7th Congress. Paraná: PED, 2006.

DATASUS. IDB. Online database, available at http://www.datasus.gov.br/idb. Access in August 2009.

DAVIM, Rejane Marie Barbosa, TORRES, Gilson de Vasconcelos, DANTAS, Susana Maria Miranda et al. Study with elderly from asylums in the municipality of Natal/RN: socioeconomic and health characteristics. Rev. Latino-Am. Enferm. [online]. May/June 2004, vol.12, no.3 p.518-524. Available at:<http://www.scielo.br/scielo.php?script=sci_arttext&pid=S0104116920 04000300010&lng=en&nrm=iso>. ISSN 0104-1169.

DESESQUELLES, Aline, BROUARD, Nicolas. Le réseau familial des personnes âgées de 60ans ou plus vivant à domicile ou en institution. Population, vol.58, n°2, 2003. p.201-227.

ELY, V. H. M. B. Ergonomics x Architecture: searching a better performance of the physical environment. In: INTERNATIONAL CONGRESS ON ERGONOMICS AND USABILITY OF HUMAN-TECHNOLOGY INTERFACES: PRODUCTS, PROGRAMS, INFORMATION,

CONSTRUCTED ENVIRONMENT, 2003, Rio de Janeiro. Congress. Rio de Janeiro: [s.n.], 2003.

FABRÍCIO, S. C. C; RODRIGUES, R. A. P.; COSTA JUNIOR, M. L. Causas e consequências de quedas de idosos atendidos em hospital público. Rev Saúde Pública, São Paulo, v.38, p. 93-99, 2004.

FABRÍCIO, S. C. C; RODRIGUES, R. A. P.; COSTA JUNIOR, M. L. Causas e consequências de quedas de idosos atendidos em hospital público. Rev Saúde Pública, São Paulo, v.38, p. 93-99, 2004.

FERNANDES, Maria Goretti ET AL. Special Topics in Worker's Health and Ergonomics. Recife: Fundação Antônio dos Santos Abranches. 2009.

FRANÇA, I. S. X.; PAGLIUCA, L. M. F.; BAPTISTA, R. S. Política de inclusão do portador de deficiência: possibilidades e limites. Acta Paul Enferm., São Paulo, v. 21, n. 1 p. 112-6, 2008.

FREITAS MC, MARUYAMA SAT, FERREIRA TF, MOTTA AMA. Perspectivas das pesquisas em gerontologia e geriatria: revisão da literatura. Rev Latino-am Enfermagem 2002 march-april; 10(2):221-8.

GIBSON, M.J., GREGORY, S. R., PANDYA, S.M. Long-term care in developed nations: a brief review. Washington, D.C.: AARP Public Policy Institute, 2003. 34p

GONÇALVES, L. G. et al. Prevalência de quedas em idosos asilados do município de Rio Grande do Sul. Rev. Saúde Pública, São Paulo, v. 42, n. 5, p. 938-45, oct. 2008.

GROISMAN, D. Old people's homes: past and present. Interdisciplinary studies on ageing 1999; 2: 67-87.

GUCCIONE, A. A. Fisioterapia Geriátrica. 2. ed. Rio de Janeiro: Guanabara Koogan, 2002.

GUIMARÃES, B. L.; OLIVEIRA, R.; MORAES, A. Diagnose ergonômica em cozinha para idosos. Rio de Janeiro: [s.n., s.d.]. Available at: <http://www.portaldoenvelhecimento.net/download/ergoidoso.pdf>. Accessed on: 11 Feb. 2009.

HAREVEN, Tamara K. Aging and Generational Relations: A Historical and Life Course Perspective. Annual Review of Sociology, Vol. 20, 1994. pp. 437-461

IBGE. Demographic Census 2000. Rio de Janeiro (RJ): Brazilian Institute of Geography and

Statistics; 2000.

IBGE. Síntese de Indicadores Sociais 2008. Available at www.ibge.gov.br. Accessed July 2009.

IIDA, I. Ergonomia Projeto e Produção. 7. reim. São Paulo: Edgard, 2001.

BRAZILIAN INSTITUTE OF GEOGRAPHY AND STATISTICS. IBGE. Preliminary data on population in Brazil. Rio de Janeiro, 2002.

KITCHENER, Martin; HARRINGTON, Charlene. The U.S. Long-Term Care Field: A Dialectic Analysis of Institution Dynamics. Journal of Health and Social LAMAS, José Manuel Ressano Garcia.Morfologia Urbana e Desenho da Cidade: 4ª Port Edition, 2007.

LAMURA, Giovanni et al. Family Carers' Experiences Using Support Services in Europe: Empirical Evidence From the EUROFAMCARE Study. The Gerontologist.

Washington,USA: The Gerontological Society of America, 2008.Vol. 48, No. 6, 752771.

LLOYD-SHERLOCK, Peter (eds). Ageing, development and Social Protection - Generalisations, Myths and Stereotypes. In: Living Longer: ageing, development and social protection.London/New York: United Nations Research Institute for Social Development/ ZED Books, 2004. 308 p.

LOUZÃ, MR NETTO; LOUZÃ, SPR; COHEN C; LOUZÃ JR. The elderly, total institutions and institutionalization. Rev Paul Hosp 1986 July-August; 34(7/8//9):135-43.

MACIEL, M. R. C. Portadores de Deficiência: a questão da inclusão social. São Paulo em Perspectiva, São Paulo, v. 14, n. 2,p. 51-56, 2006.

MARTINS, S. B. ; CANTO, S. E. . Avaliação das condições de usabilidade e acessibilidade de uma residência para idosos. In: CONGRESSO LATINO

AMERICAN CONGRESS OF ERGONOMICS. VI congress... Porto Alegre : UFRGS/PPGEP, 2001. v. 1, p. 1-13.

MARX, Roberto Burle.Arte & Paisagem:2ª Edition São Paulo: Editora Studio Nobel, 2004.

MCCULLOUGH, Laurence B. *Long-Term Care Ethics.* Encyclopedia of Aging. The Gale Group Inc. 2002. *Encyclopedia.com.* http://www.encyclopedia.com Accessed May 5, 2009.

MATSUDO, S. M.; MATSUDO, V. K. R.; NETO, T. L. B. Impacto do envelhecimento nas variáveis antropométricas, neuromotoras e metabólicas da aptidão física. Rev. Bras. Ciên.

e Mov., Brasília, v.8, n.4, p.21-32, sep. 2000.

MATURANA, R. , CARBONELL, C. G. Pacientes amputados: Adaptación Psicosocial. Salud Mental, Santiago,.v. 42, n.1 , p. 40-44, dec, 1999.

MEANS, K.M., RODELL, D.E.; O'SULLIVAN, P.S. Use of an obstacle course to assess balance and mobility in the elderly: a validation study. Am J Phys Med Rehabil, [S.I.], v. 75, n. 2, p. 88-95, 1996.

MEDEIROS, M.; DINIZ, D. Aging and Disability: Internaional Classification of Functioning Disability and Health (ICIDH-2). Geneva: [s.n.], 2001.

MOREIRA, M. M. S. Trabalho, qualidade de vida e envelhecimento. 2000. 91f. Dissertation (Master in Public Health) - Center for the Study of Worker's Health and Human Ecology, Oswaldo Cruz Foundation, Rio de Janeiro, 2000.

MORENO, A; VERAS, R. O idoso e as instituições asilares no município do Rio de Janeiro. Gerontologia 1999; 7 (4): 167-77.

MUNIZ, M. M. B. R. Acessibilidade: questão de cidadania. Revista Reviva, Brasília, year 2, p. 53-54, 2005.

NAKAMURA, E. K. K. O trabalho de pessoas com restrições oriundas de deficiências em instituições bancárias. Florianópolis, 2003. 198f. Thesis (Doctorate in Production Engineering) - Universidade Federal de Santa Catarina - UFSC, Santa Catarina, 2003.

NÉRI, AL. As políticas de atendimento aos direitos da pessoa idosa expressam no Estatuto do Idoso. A Terceira Idade, v.16, n.34, p.7-24, 2005.

NEUFERT, Ernst. The Art of Designing in Architecture. São Paulo: Gustavo Gili, do Brasil, 2009.

UNITED NATIONS ORGANIZATION, UN. Second World Assembly on Ageing, 2002. http://www.

un.orgZesaZsocdevZ

ageingZsecondworld02.htmlconsulta in

December 2007.

PARAHYBA, M.I. VERAS, R. Sociodemographic differentials in functional decline in physical mobility among the elderly in Brazil. Revista Ciência e saúde Coletiva, Rio de Janeiro, v.13, n.004, p.1257-1264, jul-ag, 2008.

PEREIRA, M. C.; FERNANDES, M. G.; SANTOS, M. A. Intervenções ergonómicas nos postos de trabalho para portadores de necessidades especiais - artigo de revisão. 2007. 15f. Course Conclusion Work (Graduação) - UNICAP, Recife, 2007.

PEREIRA, S. R. M. et al Quedas em Idosos: projeto diretrizes. Rio de Janeiro: Sociedade Brasileira de Geriatria e Gerontologia, 2001. Available at: http://www.projetodiretrizes.org.br/projeto_diretrizes/082.pdf. Accessed on: 04 Apr. 09.

QUALHARINI, E. L.; ANJOS, F. C. Ergonomia do espaço edificado para pessoas portadoras de deficiência: o projeto sem barreiras. 1. ed. Niteroi: Universidade Federal Fluminense, 1997.

RIBEIRO, A. P. et al The influence of falls on the quality of life of the elderly. Ciênc. Saúde Coletiva. Rio de Janeiro, v. 13, n. 4, p. 1265-73, aug. 2008.

ROLIM, Marcos. Between silence and death. Available at <http://www.rolim.com.br/2002/modules.php?name=Sections&sop=viewarticle&artid= 48>created in March 2002, accessed 10/09/2005

SÁ, F. D et al. Ergonomic adaptations and balance in elderly: descriptive analysis of the risk of falls in a long-stay institution in João Pessoa, Paraíba. In: ENEGEP, 26, 2006, Fortaleza. XXVI ENEGEP. Fortaleza, ABEPRO, 2006.

SANCHES, ARP. Santa Catarina Retirement Home. Available at: http://www.casasderepouso.org/casaderepouso-27.html. Casa de repouso sta Catarina. Accessed on: 22 April 2010.

SANTOS, A.; SANTOS, L. K. S.; RIBAS, V. G. Acessibilidade de habitações de interesse social ao cadeirante: um estudo de caso. Ambiente Construído, [S.l.], v. 5, n. 1, p. 55-75. jan./mar., 2005.

SANTOS, C.L.M.e ANDRADE, C.M. Incidência de quedas relacionada aos fatores de risco em idosos institucionalizados. Revista Baiana de Saúde Pública vol. 29 p.57-68 January 2005.

SANTOS, M. L. C. ; ANDRADE, M. C. Incidência de Quedas relacionada aos fatores de riscos em idosos institucionalizados. Revista Baiana de Saúde Pública, Salvador. v. 29, n. 1, p. 57-68, 2005.

SANTOS, Mauro; BURSZTYN, Ivani (rg.). Saúde e Arquitetura - Caminhos para a humanização dos Ambientes Hospitalares. Rio de Janeiro: Editora SENAC, 2004.Saúde

Pública, São Paulo, v. 33, n. 5, p. 445-453. Oct. 1999.

SBGG (Sociedade Brasileira de Geriatria e Gerontologia - São Paulo Section) - Instituição de Longa Permanência para Idosos: manual de funcionamento. São Paulo, Brazilian Society of Geriatrics and Gerontology - São Paulo Section, 2003:39 p.

SILBAUGH, Katharine. The Structures of Care Work. Chicago-Kent Law Review, 2001, vol. 76. pp.1389-1402.

SOARES, M. M. Ergonomics and Design: an interaction to be intensified. [S.n.t.] Disponívelem   :
<http://www.construccion.uniovi.es/ergonomia/congresos/2005/ergonomia/industrial. pdf>. Accessed on: 15 feb. 2009.

SONN, U.; GRIMBW, G. and SVANBORG, A. Activities of daily living studied longitudinally between 70 and 76 years of age. Disabil Rehabil., [S.l.], v. 18, n. 2, p. 91-100, 1996.

SOUSA L, GALANTE H, FIGUEIREDO D. Qualidade de vida e bem-estar dos idosos: um estudo exploratório na população portuguesa. Rev Saúde Pública 2003 June; 37(3):364-71.

STAMATO, C. ; MORAIS, A. A visão de idosos cariocas sobre a segurança do banheiro domiciliar. In: INTERNATIONAL CONGRESS ON DESING RESEARCH IN BRAZIL. 4° congress... Rio de Janeiro. [s.n.], 2007.

TELLECHEA, Lourdes. Cuidados permanentes de las personas mayores. Paper presented at the Meeting of Governments and Experts on Ageing in South American Countries. Buenos Aires, Argentina: 14-16 November 2005, available at http:ZZwww.eclac.clZceladeZnoticiasZpaginasZ4Z23004ZLTellechea_d.pdf

TOMÉ, C. A.; MÁSCULO, F.S. Avaliação Ergonómica do Ambiente Construído: Asylums. Ergonomic Evaluation of the Built Environment: Asilos. In: CONGRESSO

BRASILEIRO DE ERGONOMIA, 14., 2006, Curitiba. 14° congress... Curitiba: ABERGO, 2006.

VASCONCNCELOS, D. T.; FERNANDES, M. G.; SIQUEIRA, G. R. Acessibilidade para portadores de necessidades especiais na clinica escola de instituição de ensino superior particular em recife/PE. 2008. Course Conclusion Work (Graduação) - Faculdade Integrada do Recife, 2008.

VASCONCELOS, T. C.; FERNANDES, M. G. O uso da ergonomia e da acessibilidade na inserção de trabalhadores com necessidades especiais na empresa - artigo de revisão. 2008. 12f.Trabalho de Conclusão de Curso (Graduation Coursework) - Faculdade Integrada do Recife, Recife, 2008.

VELOZ, M. C. T ; NACIMENTO, S.; CAMARGO, B. V. Representações sociais do envelhecimento. Psicol. Reflex. Crit., Rio de Janeiro, v.12, n.2, 1999.

VELOZ, Maria Cristina Triguero; NASCIMENTO-SCHULZE, Clélia Maria; CAMARGO, Brigido Vizeu. Social representations of aging. Psicol. Reflex. Crit. Porto Alegre, v.12, n.2, 1999. Available at: http://www.scielo.br/scielo.php?script=sci_arttext&pid=S010279721999000200015&lng=en&nrm=iso>.

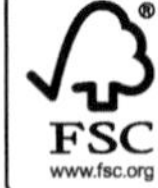